*To my Mother, who showed me how
to roll with the punches, facing life's challenges
with dignity and humor.*

Published 2018 by Gildan Media LLC
aka G&D Media
www.GandDmedia.com

ISBN: 978-1-7225-0034-4

A woman is like a tea bag—you can't tell how strong she is until you put her in hot water.

—Eleanor Roosevelt

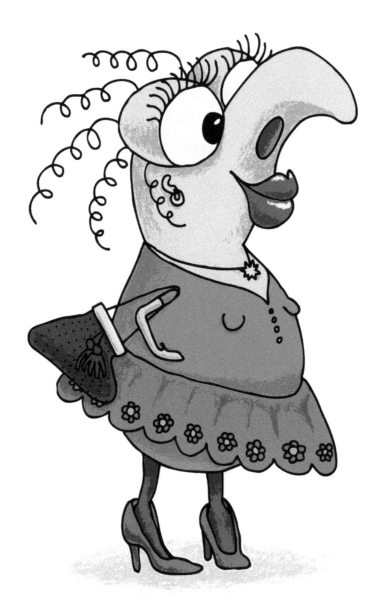

PLAYTIME AT THE ZOO

My husband's always begged me, be an animal in bed.
He's been waiting for a sex kitten
Since the night that we were wed.
Well, I've turned into an animal, and more than one or two.
In fact, I know the last I checked,

I'M QUITE A FREAKING ZOO!

I have these ugly crows feet where my blue eyes used to be.
A turkey neck's replaced the chin that always worked for me.
My legs are snakes, just shedding skin,
They flake off all day long.
And my arms have turned to bat wings,
And are shaped completely wrong!
My hair is shedding like my dog's, a little falls each day.
So come on honey, come to bed,

YOUR ANIMAL WANTS TO PLAY!

OL' BLUE EYES

I must go to the doctor. I cannot see your face,
Unless you stand so far away, you're in another place.

I never see a menu unless it's on the floor,
Or the waiter holds it in his hands,
And walks outside the door.

I guess it's not too bad this way. It's actually quite fine,

Cause I can't see your wrinkled face,
And I know you can't see mine!

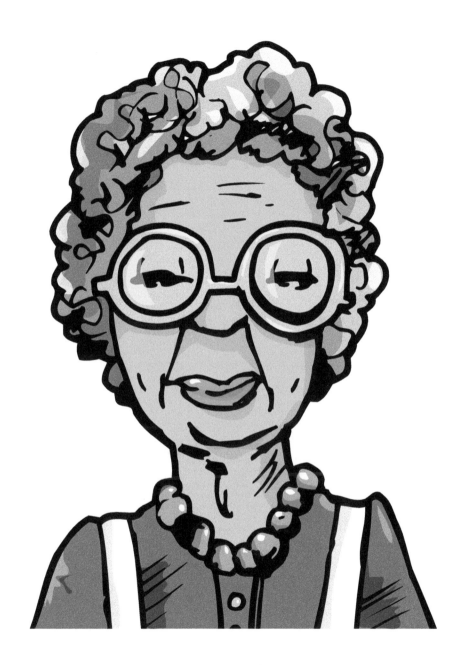

TOOTH ACHE

Don't you feel my deepest love when I smile at you?
Even though my teeth are fake, my feelings still run true.
Actually, not all are false, most teeth are half in place....
They're in caps and crowns and laminates
Just hiding in my face.

The braces I wore on my teeth to have a perfect bite,
Were such a stupid waste of time,
'Cause all moved left and right.

My teeth are overlapping.
My gums are bleeding red.

I just might have a lawsuit here,
If my orthodontist wasn't DEAD!

But for the teeth that I have left, I thank my lucky star.
I'd rather have them in my mouth than
SOAKING IN A JAR.

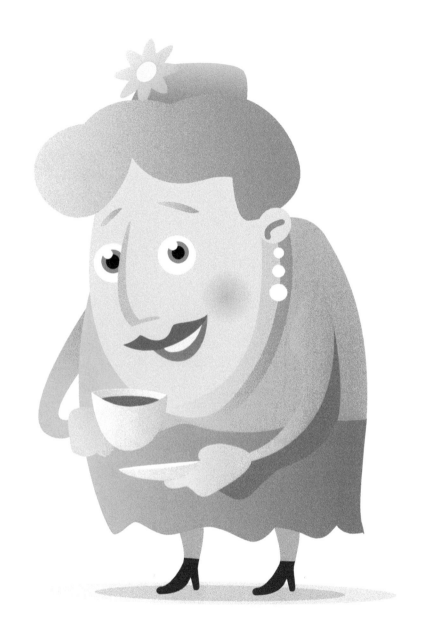

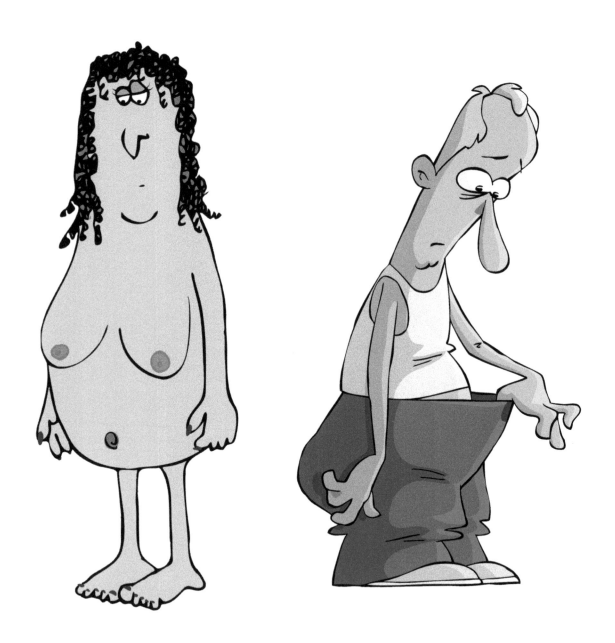

LOOK OUT BELOW!

Who discovered gravity, and where is he today?
I'd like to kill the bum that made my body fall this way!

My boobs have fallen to my knees.
My ass dropped down a flight.
My cheeks have now turned into jowls.
My eyelids block my sight!

My plumbing and my uterus too, slipped down so very far,
I fear that if I hit a bump, they'll fall out in my car!

My husband always teases me,
How low my parts have dropped.
And though his muscles still are firm,

HIS PRIVATE PART HAS FLOPP
                                    E
                                        D
                                          !

THE WEB!

My legs, my legs, my once beautiful legs,
They had been the texture of milk.
One day I was wearing the shortest of skirts,
And stockings, the sheerest of silk.

Then all of a sudden, the Spiderman hit!
He made vein webs of purple and blue!

But you won't see the lumps and the hideous bumps....

If I now only stand FACING you!

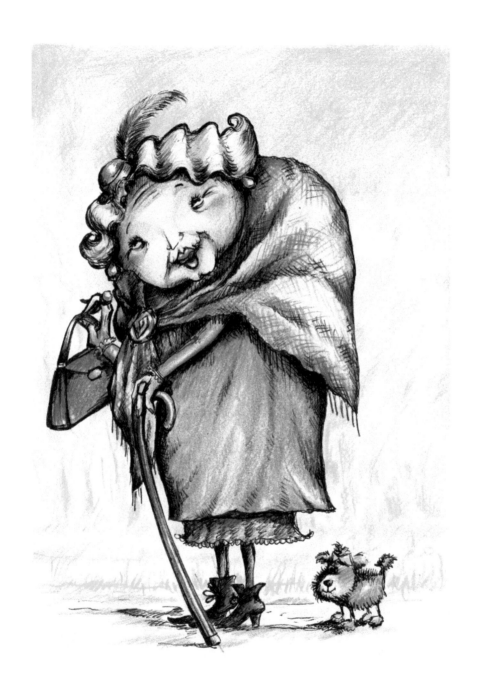

IT'S ONLY NATURAL

I have no time. I'm very late, so please dear, wish me luck.
I have to meet a special man who really knows how to tuck.

He's a wonderful plastic surgeon...
You must have heard his name.
His lifts and liposuctions have brought him tons of fame.

Collagen,
And laser beams,
And saline implants too,
All combine to help maintain,
A perfectly natural you!

So join me now and let's get fixed, and don't have any fears.
We'll pretend we're still quite young,
All through our golden years.
We'll pay him what he asks for. It's worth it just to know,
Instead of looking sixty-five,

We're each a perfect Fifty FAUX!

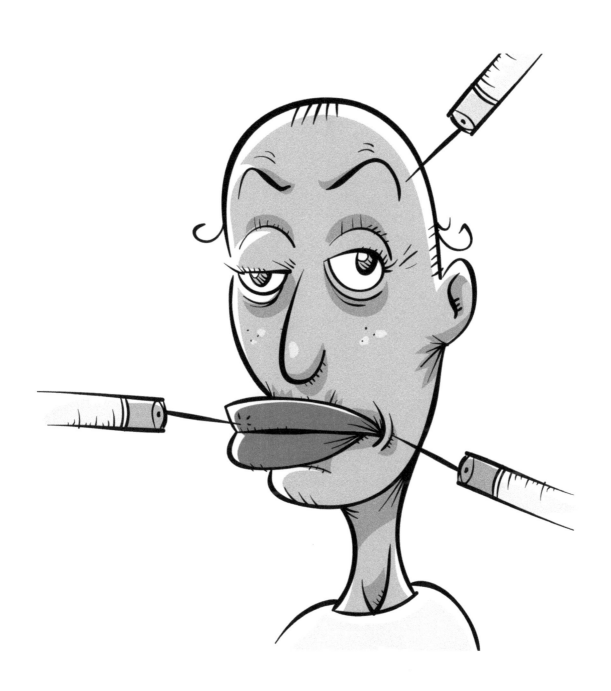

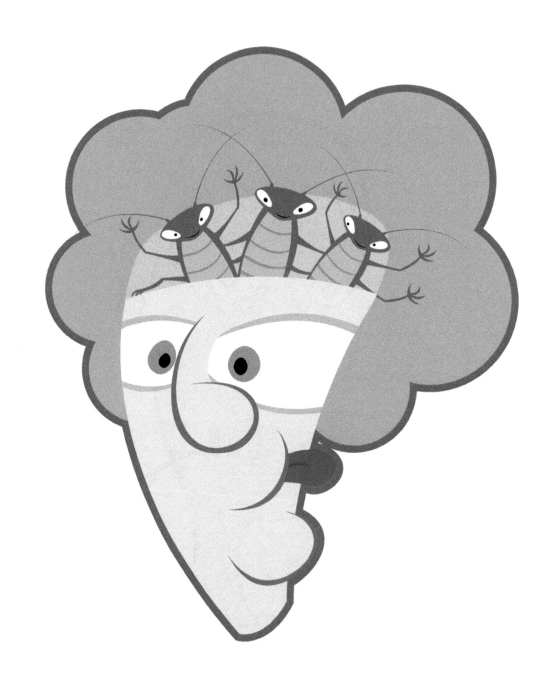

THANKS FOR THE MEMORIES

I've seen your face a hundred times.
I used to know your name,
But since I've turned this awful age,
My memory's not the same.

I forget the reason that I called.
I forget what I must do.
I know you sit there hoping,
That I'll forget I'm mad at you.

I repeat my favorite story, a dozen times or more.
But you forget you've heard it the dozen times before.
I repeat my favorite story, a dozen times or more.
Did I just say that? Yes I did, but no one's keeping score!

I think they need a telethon, or a large celebrity sing,
To raise funds for this disease called CRAFT…

CAN'T REMEMBER A FREAKING THING!

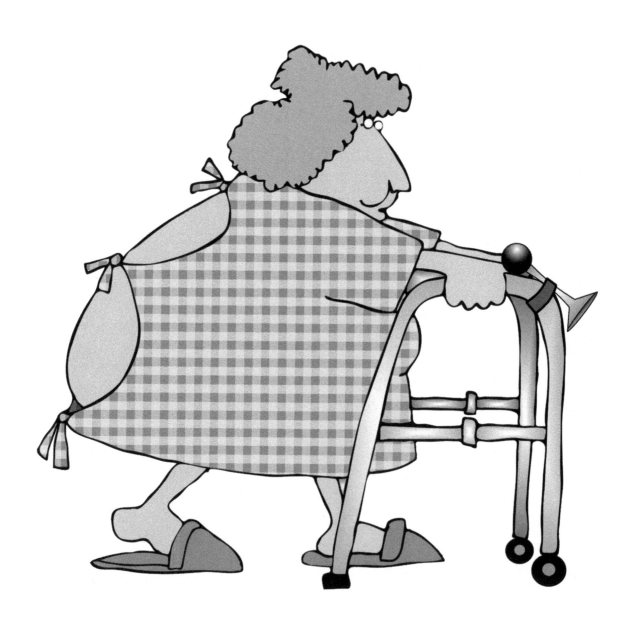

TUNE UP

I've reached the age where I'm falling apart. Every inch of my body is worn.
Fluids and mileage have piled up in me, since that beautiful day I was born.
So it's time for a tune up to check all my parts, and it's really quite a pain.
All the testing and probing and constant disrobing, is enough to drive me insane.

With much trepidation I go for a mammo. My breasts get quite a squeeze.
My dignity's gone when I visit the Gyno, and see her between my knees.
The Derm for a check of my body, never fun as I lie there quite bare.
And then for a look at my colon.
That long tube is going where?!

A shot to prevent pneumonia, and one for the shingles and flu.
A doctor to check for glaucoma. I can't hear, so they test my ears too.
I'm wired as they watch my heart rate. Lots of lines going up and then down.
I run very fast on a treadmill, in sneakers and short paper gown.

A scan of carotid, an upper GI, Drinking liquids that taste just like chalk.
So dizzy from all these appointments,
They test my balance, by watching me walk.

I've been checked head to toe, both inside and out.
For a woman my age, I still pass.

I don't want to complain, or they'll scope me again, but

THIS IS A PAIN IN THE ASS!

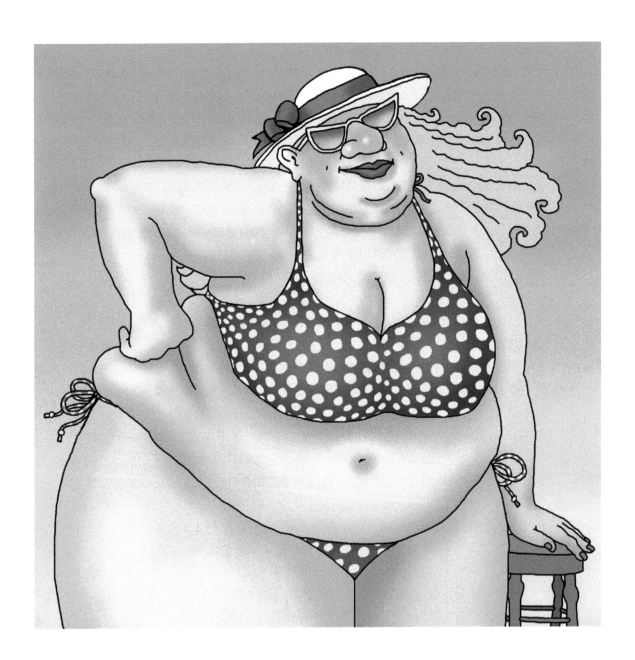

RETAINING

I look like I am pregnant,
Twelve months of the year.
My once tiny, flattened tummy
Is forever gone, I fear.

It used to be that once a month,
For seven days I'd bloat.

Now every day throughout the year…

I'm big enough to float!

FIREWORKS

Who turned off the air conditioning?
Who turned on the heat?
It feels as though I'm slowly cooking like a slab of meat!
I wake up in a sweat at night, wet and dripping hair.
All my sheets and pillows drenched, as if you really care!

You tell me that it isn't hot. It seems just right to you.
Well I know that my face is flushed,
And you haven't got a clue!

I feel the heat go up my neck. My armpits drip with sweat.
My hands have gotten clammy.
And my clothes are soaking wet!

I know what you're doing…

You're playing with my head!

BUT IF YOU TOUCH THAT HEAT AGAIN,
YOU'LL WISH THAT YOU WERE DEAD!

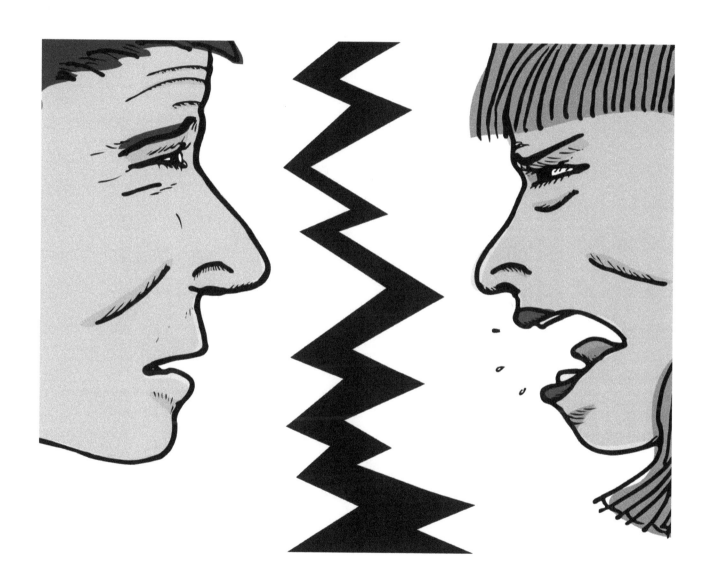

BLUE BLOODS

My skin is getting dry and thin.
I see my veins right through.
My body's like a roadmap
Of vessels, thick and blue.

Another ugly part of aging.
I'll just add it to the list.
At least they won't be hard to find,
If I decide to slit my wrist!

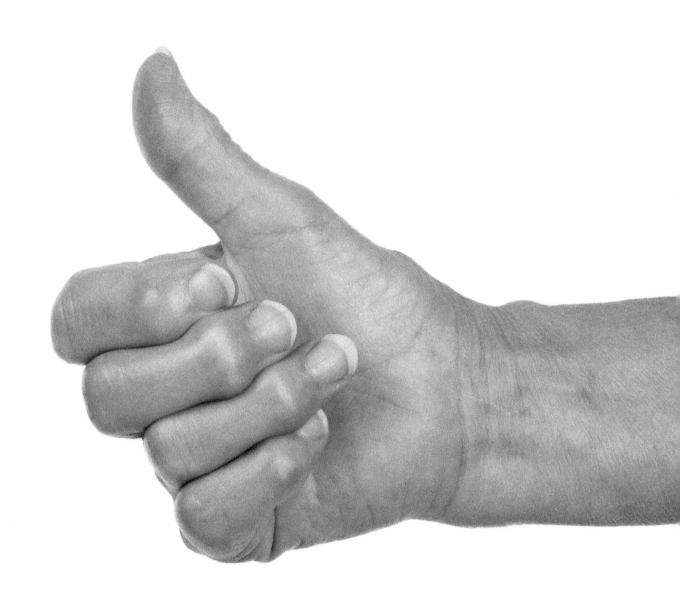

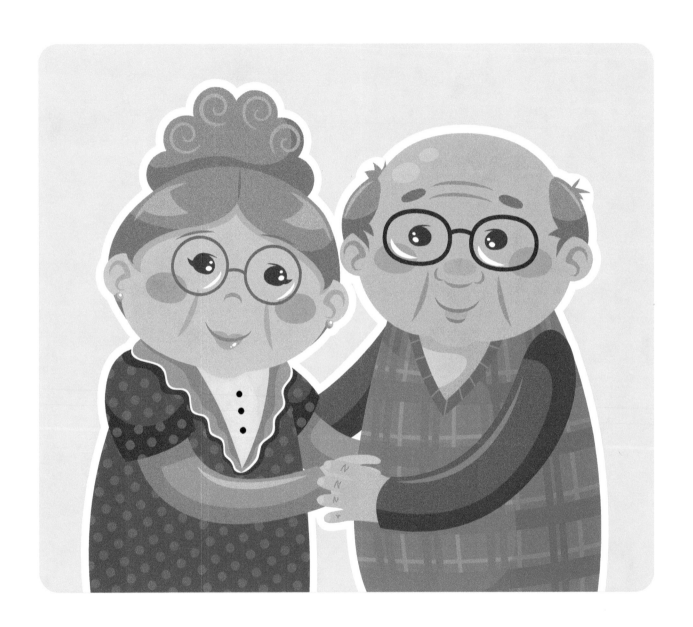

FUZZY WUZZY

I'm having a nervous breakdown here.
I can't get ahead of the grey.
I used to pull out a couple of hairs,
But now dozens come in every day!
They feel like they're made up of wire and frizz.
They make my whole hairdo look shoddy.
They look like the hair that already grows
On another part of my body.

I've tried to cover them every which way.
I've used levels 1, 2 and 3.
But the color keeps changing with every shampoo,
So I'm not even sure, this is me!

I used to tweeze my eyebrows, and one hair, here or there,
But lately I just can't keep up…they're sprouting everywhere!
Upset and quite embarrassed, I cried real salty tears,
Until I saw my husband

GROWING HAIR INSIDE HIS EARS!

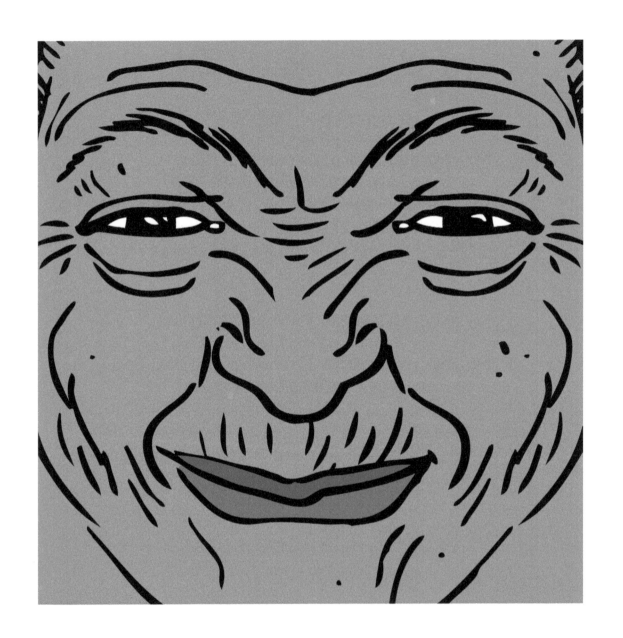

SPOTLIGHT

Out! Out! Damn Spots all over my face,
On my hands and my legs, and most every place.

I've tried bleaches and fade creams, and that strong Retin-A.
I've tried peeling and scraping them, day after day.

An acid that burns a hole in your floor,
Won't take out a liver spot.
Each day I grow more!

I think that the way to rid each small dot,
Is to bake in the sun,

'Til I'm one huge tan spot!

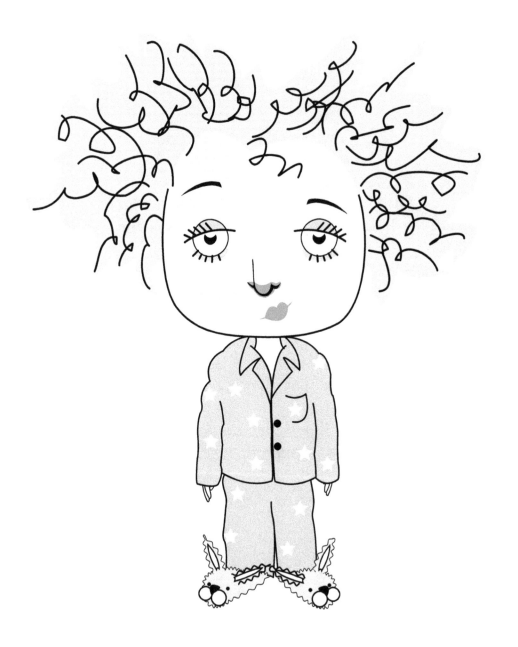

SLEEPLESS

I haven't slept in many years, I just stare at the wall.
And if per chance I start to doze, my bladder gives a call.
I toss and turn, kick off the sheets,
And count sheep 'til I'm blue.
I cannot find a comfy spot, not even next to you.

So stay there on the other side.
Don't try to cuddle me.
I'm in no mood to be disturbed,
So please, just let me be.

Yes, I'm cranky, you'd be, too, if you never fell asleep,
But you doze off without a hitch, you rested, happy, creep!

WHOOSH!

I think that I am jet propelled, I've so much gas inside.
Why, you could harness what I've got,
And you'd have quite a ride.

No matter what I eat or drink, I gurgle through the day.
I think this indigestion, is really here to stay.

Can't have acids. Can't have greens.
Can't eat too much meat.
I stay away from fatty foods, and that gooey chocolate treat.

I won't have any spicy meal, then take a ride with you,
'Cause you will have to hold your breath
Until you turn quite blue!

I've given up caffeine and booze, and beans, and even soup.
But now and then I let one go that spins me in a loop!

So if you have to sit by me, be sure you're anchored down.

I'm known to pass the strongest gas of anyone in town.

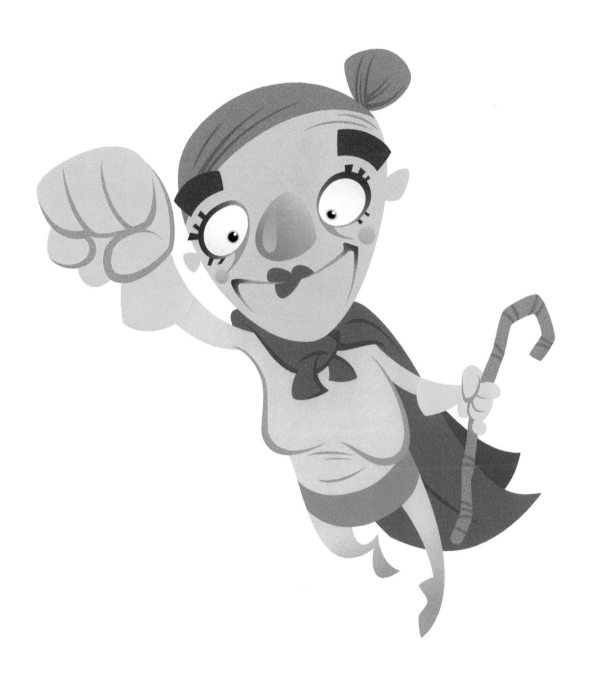

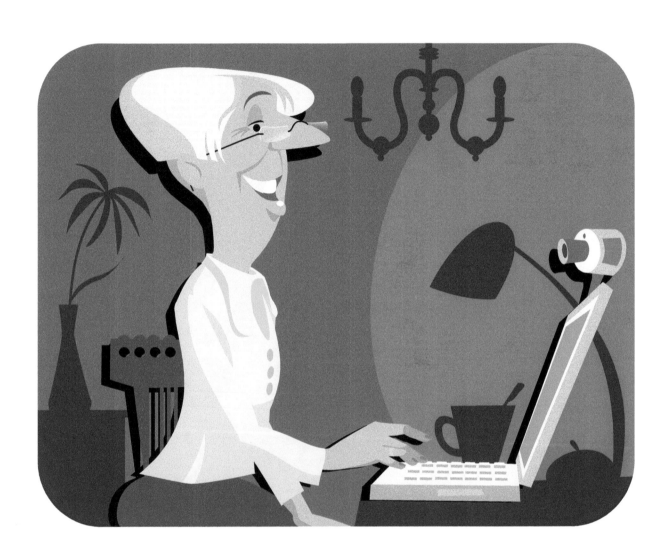

GOOD WORK!

I went to get a job last week
And it was going well,
Until the dreaded question…
Please don't make me tell!

He said he had to do a check
And asked for my birth date.
I told him it was very close
To nineteen forty-eight.

He said that I was much too old,
And he wouldn't hire me.
So I left and called my husband…
And he bought the company.

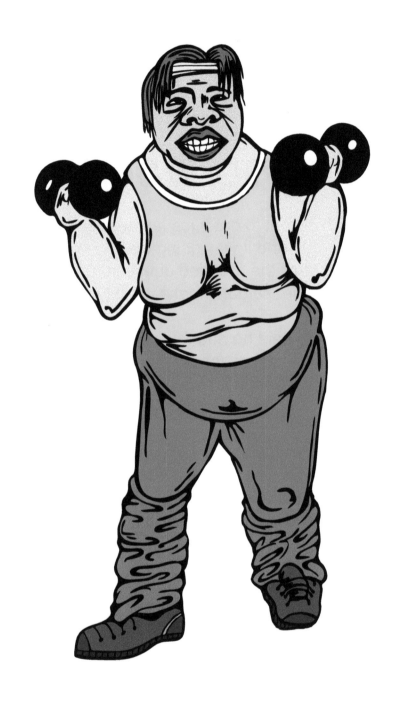

MUFFINS AND BUNS

Muffins and buns, muffins and buns!
Would you all like some muffins and buns?

They're something quite new, never had them before,
'though I still weigh the same....only 124.
But whatever I wear, I can't hold them down.
They pop up from my pants, and spread out all around.
I can suck in my breath. I can stand up real tall.
But the minute I move, they pop out, one and all!

I can run on the treadmill, take Zumba all day,
Lift weights and do sit-ups, but they're here to stay.

There's a time in the morning, just before dawn,
If I lie very still, I think "They are gone!"
I rush to my closet, and zip up my jeans.
For that second I know, what true happiness means.

But it doesn't last long. Soon reality comes,
And I'm back popping out my Muffins and Buns!

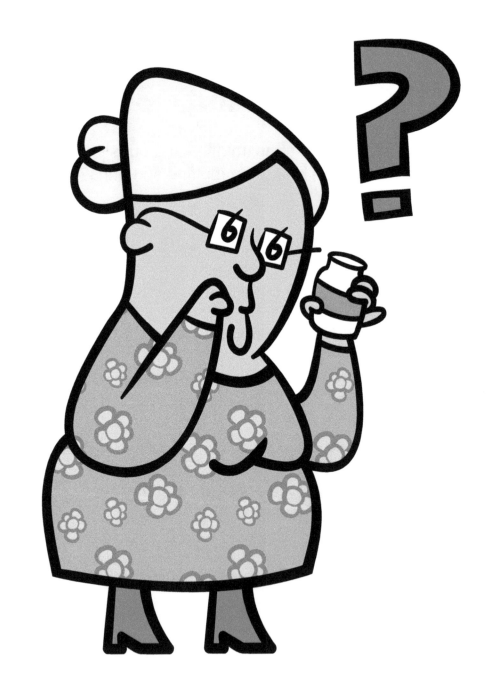

USER

I need to make a drug run to pick up all my pills.
There's one for every part of me, made just to cure my ills.
My bad cholesterol is rising, my hormone level's down.
I have the biggest mood swings, of anyone in town.
My mitral valve is acting up, blood pressure though, is good.
I hate to take my vitamins, but the doctor said I should.

A pill to help digest my food, an aspirin for my heart.
And then a little estrogen, that's for a private part.
There's calcium for loss of bone, so I won't break a hip.
And something for the pimple that has formed above my lip.
Magnesium, and Flax Seeds, and of course, Omega 3,
Black Cohosh to reduce night sweats,
And a pill to help me pee.
Some ambien if I must sleep, and a pill to calm me down.
I meet my dealer every month at the pharmacy in town.

SHRINKAGE

I used to be a full five foot four.
Now I'm five foot three.
But I don't remember cutting off any part of me.

When did it happen? How could it be?
Where did part of me go?
I think I'm all here. I still look the same,
From my head down to my toe.

My body is shrinking right into itself.
It's hard now to stand straight and tall.
But taking Pilates is just too much work.

So I'm shorter…

To hell with it all!

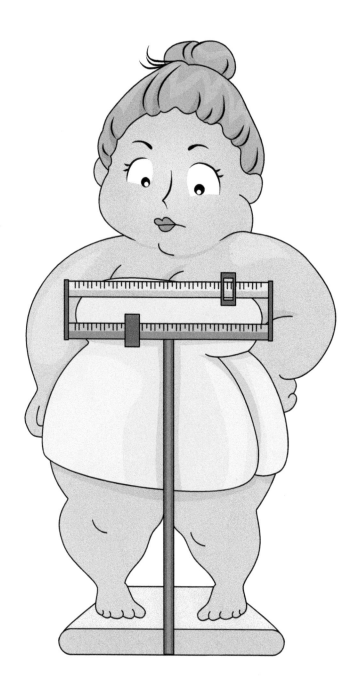

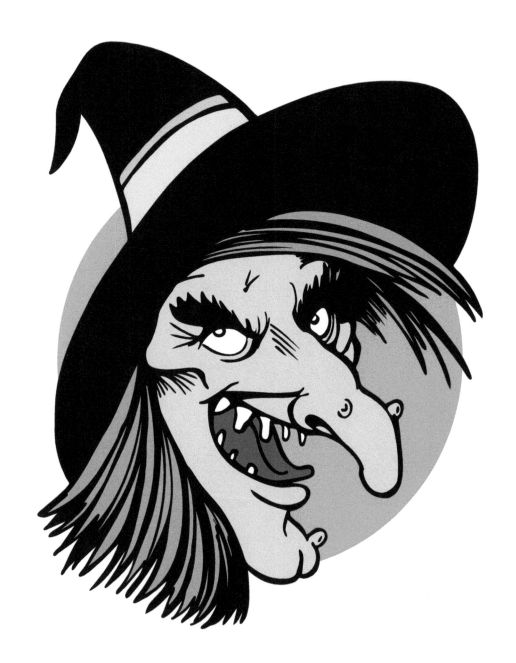

CRACKLES

Remember the days, watching cereal pop
As soon as you'd pour the milk in?
Well now it takes only, a day more of aging,
To have things pop up on your skin.

Each skin tag the size of a Krispie,
They make tons of money for Docs.
You can leave them alone,
And pretend they're not there,
But it looks like a case of the Pox.

So you have them removed, and the very next day,
You look in the mirror and then...
What a surprise, there's one under your eye.
Yes, your face is snap, crackling again!

POP!

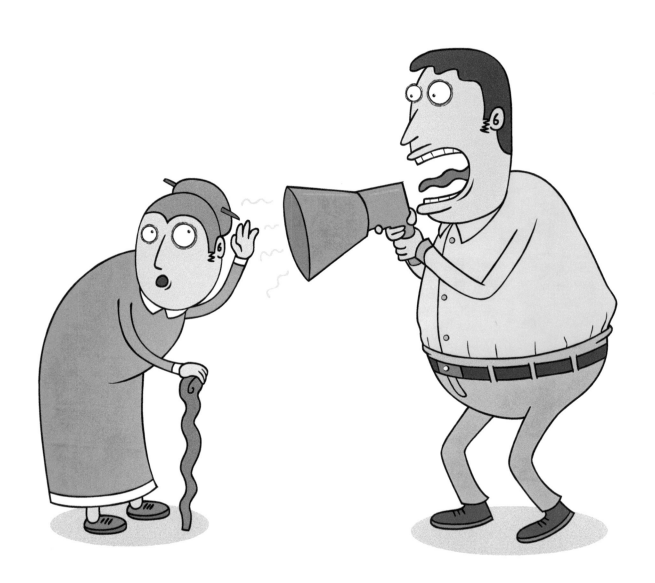

CAN YOU HEAR ME NOW?

What's happened to my eardrums?
They used to work so well.
Why, I could hear most every word
From a whisper to a yell.
I'd hear my babies in their cribs from 200 yards away.
Now I'm lucky, if I hear, every OTHER word they say.

But maybe this is not so bad,
Because when my grown kids call,
I only hear the things I want,
And they have no clue, at all!

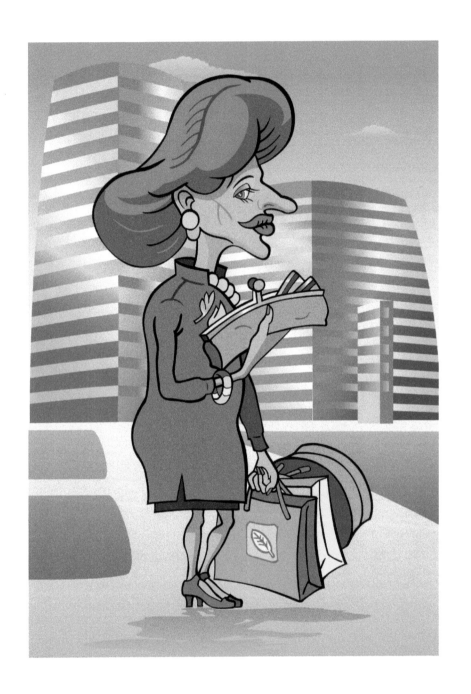

SERIOUSLY?

I used to wear the coolest clothes. I'd strut right down the street.
My shoes all had the highest heels, and looked great on my feet.
It's hard to be in vogue now, and it makes me very sad,
That my body doesn't fit at all, into the latest fad.

The pants have gotten lower, as my waist has gotten thick,
So even if I get them on, the sight would make you sick.
The heels have gotten higher, but my tendons just won't stretch.
And those ugly, painful bunions, are enough to make you retch!

The shorts are like the ones I wore, on legs once smooth and sleek.
Now they're bumpy, spotted, veiny,
And not the look I seek.

And let's discuss those handbags, that weigh 10 pounds or more.
I love the hardware and the style, but can't lift them off the floor.

Who's designing clothes for me? I'm really in between.
I won't dress like my mother, and I can't dress like a teen.
I want to wear the latest styles, but they are hard to find.

There are no super cool jeans,
That will cover my behind!

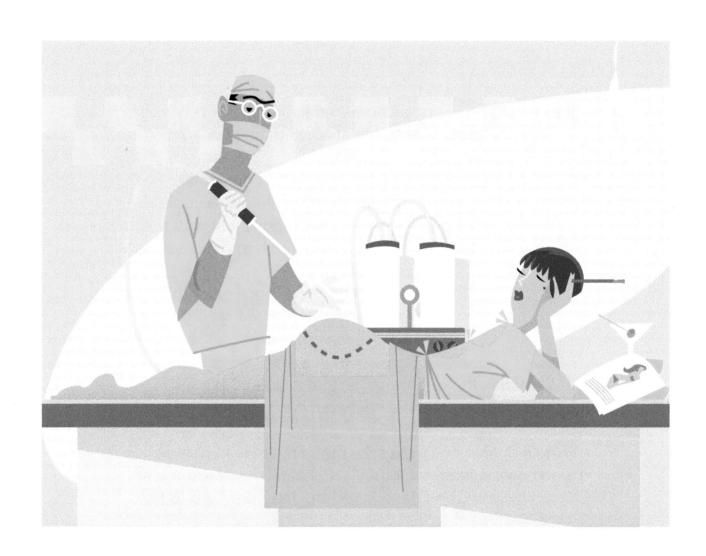

PARTS DEPARTMENT

Marsha got a brand new knee. Caren got a hip.
Collagen gave Susan Shay a brand new pouty lip.

Lucy's fat was moved a bit, from her ass up to her face.
And Frannie's doctor put her eyebrows in another place.

Alma had a real pig valve, put inside her heart.
Implants went in Susie's mouth, when her old teeth fell apart.

Carol had her breasts moved up;
Her stomach fat sucked out.
And Joan's old head has a brand new neck...
Of that there is no doubt.

Yes, we're being held together
And we're marching straight ahead.
We'll stand and fight for our new parts...

Until pronounced, officially DEAD!

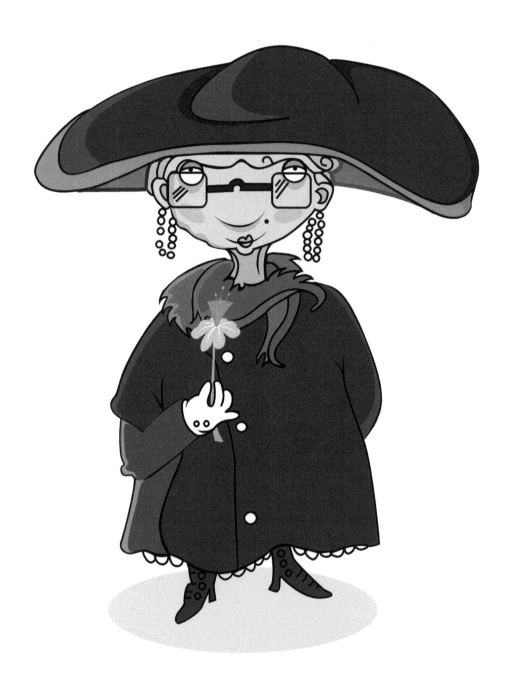

GRATEFUL

As women we may bitch a lot,
But the thing that makes us great,
Is we are there for one another,
And don't trust all things to fate.

We are the generation, that's not the "Me! Me! Me!"
Our values are the very best,
And what's good in life, we see.

We complain about our age,
But know we're lucky to be here.
We appreciate our many friends,
Those gone, we still hold dear.

We are capable, intelligent, and our priorities are right.
We make sure to count our blessings, each and every night.

So laugh about the things you can,
And know you're not alone.

I hope the part that's last to go is your funny bone.

ABOUT THE AUTHOR

A native New Yorker, Ellen grew up in Ohio, then
moved to New Jersey with her husband, where
she taught 2nd grade until the birth of her 2 sons.
A stay-at-home mom, volunteer, founder, and officer
of various charities and organizations, Ellen was often
asked to write roasts and toasts for friends and
family members for their special occasions.
She began a career in publishing and copywriting after
raising her sons and moving to Manhattan.
An avid traveler, theatergoer, food enthusiast, and grandmother of 3 beautiful girls,
Ellen still thinks she's 40,
and makes it a point to stay away from mirrors.

"There is a fountain of youth: it is your mind, your talents,
the creativity you bring to your life and the lives of people you love.
When you learn to tap this source,
you will truly have defeated age."

—Sophia Loren

Printed in the USA
CPSIA information can be obtained
at www.ICGtesting.com
JSHW072027140824
68134JS00042B/3817

9 781722 500344